Cover design or artwork by Alchemy Consulting

Order this book online at www.trafford.com/07-2189
or email orders@trafford.com

Most Trafford titles are also available at major online book retailers.

Note for Librarians: A cataloguing record for this book is available from Library and Archives Canada at www.collectionscanada.ca/amicus/index-e.html

ISBN: 978-1-4251-5039-6

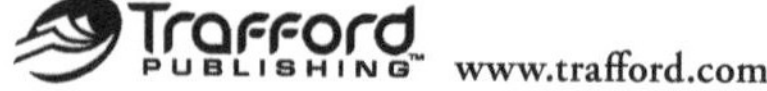

www.trafford.com

North America & international
toll-free: 1 888 232 4444 (USA & Canada)
phone: 250 383 6864 • fax: 250 383 6804 • email: info@trafford.com

The United Kingdom & Europe
phone: +44 (0)1865 722 113 • local rate: 0845 230 9601
facsimile: +44 (0)1865 722 868 • email: info.uk@trafford.com

10 9 8 7 6 5 4 3

Light + Hypnosis = ☺

DEDICATION

This book is dedicated to my departed Lakeland terrier, Duca.

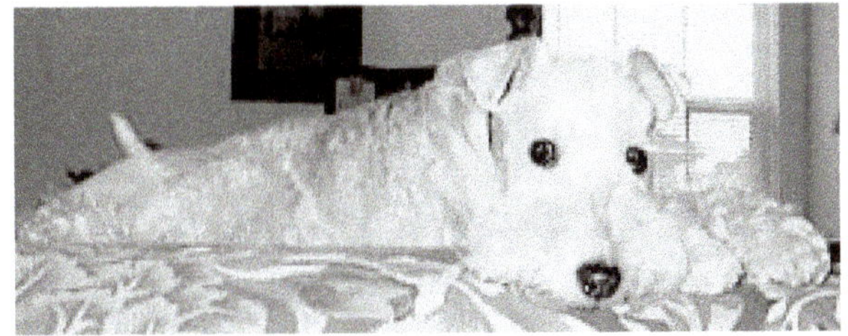

You brightened the darkest days

and showed me how to truly bask in the light.

You were so darned cute!

Your tail wagged even while you slept.

ACKNOWLEDGMENTS

I'd like to acknowledge Dr. Norman Rosenthal for his work in the area of the winter blues and St. John's Wort; Dr. Peter Kaplan, who led me to investigate the power of vitamin D; Dr. Jacob Liberman and the many other unnamed pioneers of light therapy. I'd like to acknowledge the folks at the Hypnosis Motivation Institute; Laurel Mellin for her many insights on the emotional sources of eating and their relation to cravings; and to those who crafted the lyrics presented throughout this work.

I'd like to acknowledge one very special person who allowed me the time to retest my ideas while she was also being truly challenged indeed. Lorice, you rock!

TABLE OF CONTENTS

INTRODUCTION

'Since the days of revelation, in fact, the same four corrupting errors have been made over and over again; submission to faulty and unworthy authority; submission to what it was customary to believe; submission to the prejudices of the mob; and worst of all, concealment of ignorance by a false show of unheld knowledge, for no better reason than Pride.'

Roger Bacon

This, as a first published work, is really my second attempt to 'give back' to a community of people affected by seasonal light variation, although in a less than anonymous fashion than my first. It is a rather brief work, if I may say so myself. I've been criticized by some of my friends and rather correctly I might add, as being 'terse'. I like to think of my style as similar to that of officer Joe Friday, portrayed by Jack Webb in Dragnet, who would frequently reminded the feminine subject of his interrogation to provide, 'just the facts ma'am'.

It's really a treatise on reframing one's thoughts surrounding seasonal affective disorder and how to effectively form new habits to overcome the effects of seasonal light variation.

I want you to obtain all you need to know as quick as possible so you get back to doing what's most important in your life at your maximum level of effectiveness. Along the way we'll take a few segues but I'll attempt to keep them relatively brief as I offer up my experiences in the hope that they may help you understand yours. As we go along, I'll offer up links to additional information that can be obtained from the appendix of this book and at the **Light of Day** website (http://www.ldima.com).

I began this endeavor with much greater anonymity a few years ago by running an email group on Yahoo for Seasonal Affective Disorder. I was more susceptible back then, helpless really, and didn't have a clue what to do about it. I knew one thing; I definitely wasn't alone in my struggle. I began trolling for real life experiences and offering what I had tried in exchange for something from others who had or were experiencing similar or different issues, always with an eye out for relief. I was looking for the 'cure'. Along the way I learned a thing or two and developed a response to what I have come to call 'light deprivation', that is almost as good. I want to share it with you. Please accept this body of work with an open mind.

The fact that you are reading this now tells me that you are not an ordinary person. You have a healthy self-interest in that you are searching for reasons as to why your level of effectiveness has lessened. Maybe you, like myself, often find yourself in a real funk during the winter or during an extended run of cloudy, dreary days. If so, you are on the right path. Your efforts may soon be rewarded. It just takes a little action.

Most everyone wants to make the best use of their time; they want to feel at their best, all year long. The malady that has come to be known as Seasonal Affective Disorder interferes with that process by turning some otherwise capable and effective people into dreadful doubters. I'm convinced that reasonable and healthy people are being misled into thinking they have a mental disorder. It simply isn't the case. You're not suffering from depression; you're susceptible to light-deprivation.

I'm so confident about sharing what I've come to know as true that it's time for me to step out from behind the curtain of anonymity. I simply am unable to contain myself anymore. I recall the day that I was speaking to my health care practitioner about SAD and I mentioned in passing to her that "I could write a book about it, I know it so well", as she filled out the prescription for my vitamin D. I knew right then I absolutely had to. There was no alternative for me as I was truly driven.

I'm hoping you'll see that I sincerely wish to share what I've learned and that I can show you how to put an end to your difficulty, however great or small that may be. For some, it is not trivial at all. There was a time when I counted myself among them.

To that end, this relatively brief work is the culmination of over half a lifetime of experiences attempting to define and remediate what it is that happens to me and to people like me each fall and throughout early to mid-winter. I am excited to share in fairly explicit detail, the most successful methodology I've come across that has the power to banish SAD symptoms completely and quickly too. May I say, sooner than you may have thought possible.

Again, this is not the cure. If you abandon your efforts during any period of susceptibility, your symptoms may return and much quicker than you'd like too, sad to say, no pun intended. If I ever do find a cure, you can bet the house, I'll be publishing an addendum. That is my promise to you.

These methods work in part because light therapy helps. But light therapy all on its own fails to address and tends to create sometimes subtle side effects for some. Depending on how far north and how light deprived you are when you begin light therapy, you may find yourself spending a great deal of time in front of the light box. This expenditure of time may leave one with the feeling (similar to that of mine at times) that there must be something else to do to 'speed' things along. If not to 'speed' things along, then at least something to make the amount of time spent in light therapy more productive.

Where light therapy alone sometimes fails to completely remediate the lack of motivation that accompanies seasonal light variation and often introduces feelings of inadequacy, from being light deprived or that you are somehow different from others, is right where hypnosis steps in to address these issues and will have a profound affect on the balance of your life. You may find that you become curious enough to incorporate the formal (via certified hypnotherapist) or informal (through the recorded or self-administered) use of hypnosis into your life.

To repeat, I believe my methods are successful because:

1. Light therapy corrects the source of the problem (receiving less than your minimum daily requirement of light)

2. Self-confidence and self-esteem hypnosis removes negative thinking and provides motivation at the proper intervals to supplement light-therapy and keeps you in front of the light

3. St. John's Wort (referred to as SJW from time to time and optional in this program, but if used…) works to remediate unwelcome feelings safely and subtly and elevates mood convincingly with few side effects, if any

If you are looking for an 'external solution' to the affect that light deprivation can have on your mind-body, this is the only way I have found success. By 'external solution', I am of course referring to an expression, coined by Laurel Mellin, author of the 'The Pathway' and proponent of a method to reach health and happiness referred to as 'The Solution', that refers to anything that is done to resolve the unwelcome feelings programmed into our neural networks that does not come from within. Please see the appendix for more information and links to Laurel's method.

I haven't found anything else that cures SAD, other than moving south. It is simple, effortless and effective. I encourage you to revisit the **Light of Day** website at http://www.ldima.com for follow-on updates.

I currently reside at latitude 40 in the northern hemisphere. Please try this method of combining hypnosis and light therapy with an open mind and I believe you will find that it will work for you too, regardless of where you reside.

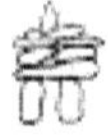

HOW DID I GET HERE?

"Sometimes I give myself the creeps
Sometimes my mind plays tricks on me
It all keeps adding up
I think I'm cracking up..."
Green Day – Basket Case

I first became aware that something was a little different about me when I was 13 years of age. From then on every fall, a feeling of dread descended upon my mood and I became increasingly anxious as the winter holidays approached. Some years the anxiety did not recede until the following March or April. But it was always gone completely by May, June at the very latest.

Some years, usually around the time of the summer solstice, I thought back to Christmas & New Years and wondered whether I had actually felt as bad as I did. This often led me to question if the susceptibility had been all in my mind. It has never ceased to amaze me, the difference in how I feel in June as compared to December.

Needless to say, these feelings aroused an amount of uncertainty that spread slowly, somewhat like a benign form of cancer, throughout my conscious and unconscious thought process. I confidently say that part of me has now been 'cured'. I no longer suffer from the uncertainty of wondering what may be 'wrong' with me. I don't have a disorder either, but I'm capable of feeling very much at 'dis-ease'.

As that youngster, I lacked a certain knowledge of myself and was yet to attain the depth of awareness adulthood brings. I often associated seasonally unwelcome feelings, whenever they occurred, with what had been going on in my life at that time, you know, the old 'cause and effect' type of thinking. This is exactly the kind of thing that neuro-linguistic programming or NLP practitioners have come to call 'anchoring'. I linked up a particular event with those feelings and wrote it off as a life experience and moved on. It eventually became an ingrained pattern of existence, wired into my neural networks and needless to say, I no longer wished to experience fall and winter.

I'd like to say that leaving my hometown was a tough decision for a kid that had grown up in snowy western New York, but the truth is that I decided rather early on to go and head further south. I felt I needed to finish school and solidify my career path first. Then I'd begin to look for the appropriate opportunity. In hindsight, it was not the optimum decision. Given the shallow depth of understanding concerning Seasonal Affective Disorder that existed at that time, the best decision may have been to head south first, ask questions later! Looking back, I will honestly say my instincts were in the right place, I simply didn't have the tools or the capacity to change.

I grew up with and experienced a consistent theme of light deprivation and it took a long time before I learned to give myself what I needed when I needed it. Out of necessity and lack of space due to the healthy-sized Catholic family that I come from, I lived in the basement of my parent's 3-bedroom home and shared a thoughtfully added-on fourth room with my younger brother. It wasn't all that bad mind you, you can get away with a lot when you don't have to waltz by your folks when you return home at night <wink, wink>. As you can imagine, it was dark all the time in the cellar too.

People who visit me nowadays sometimes remark how bright it is in my home and are amazed at how many lights I have on at any given time. This may be initially written off as an over-reaction to my earlier days of light deprivation, but I think it's not. I believe we affected individuals cannot function in a mushroom-like existence and that we must insist on our 'right to light'. No one should have to live as if they are in a cave. It simply is not healthy for us.

I know the electrical distribution charge of my monthly utility bill is usually equal to and sometimes exceeds the actual usage portion, so I don't lose sleep over the amount I'm paying for the electricity needed to brighten my life. I wish I could say the same for my natural gas usage but that's for another day. Suffice it to say that you should not notice much of a change budget-wise either when you choose to adopt my 'light-style'. The benefits far outweigh the cost.

Oh, and please think twice before converting over to compact fluorescent lighting either, it currently leaves much to be desired.

Living outside Buffalo at the time of the blizzard of '77, an indelible event that sent many people in western New York forever south, I eventually graduated from college and found a job in my chosen career, fulfilling the all-important life plan requirement. But love intervened in my life and after a few more dark and snowy winters, while in my late twenties, I eventually relocated to a slightly more southern and somewhat sunnier location in central New Jersey.

It made quite an indelible impression on me, when my mother commented on how "one could really use a good pair of sunglasses" when visiting me in my new home. With this fresh start, I left the past behind and along with it, the as then still undiscovered sources of the seasonally and quite naturally recurring events that were helping to define much of my life experience. Or so it seemed. If only it had been that simple.

I relocated in the month of June. I planned the move during the prior fall and winter. This is noteworthy. And it is so for the following reason. One of the 'markers' that you have seasonal mood tendencies is whether you find things 'happen' for you in your life during late spring and early summer. I know it's easy to say that things will happen then because the school calendar makes it easier and you become conditioned to expect things to occur at that time of the year. At the end of the day, if you find it easier to accomplish your goals in late spring and early summer, you're on to something as far as seasonal mood variation is concerned.

I want you to take a deeper dive and see whether you are able to remember how things transpired in your life with greater ease, the closer you got to the summer solstice. Take a few moments and put this book down while you think back. See if you identify a seasonal pattern to, or if any events in your life have been accomplished with ease around late June. I've left some space for you to journal below. Think about it a little and see if you can find anything accomplished with ease at the end of spring or in early summer.

1) ______________________________

____

____

2) ______________________________

____

____

3) ______________________________

____

____

The fall after my 'big' move to Jersey, I began to experience that same old feeling of dread again. I originally thought it was just pressure from my girlfriend of wanting to be married that was the real source of the dread. I suppose it's possible. But again, I come to the conclusion that it's simply another instance of the same old cause and effect way of thinking, trying to rationalize what's going on in our lives and the failure to think deeper, to find the root cause.

Two degrees of latitude separate western New York and central, NJ. When you've got the winter blues, every degree further south helps and each sunny day brings tremendous relief. Suddenly, geography and meteorology have the power to conspire for or against you, or so it seems. The less cloudy the weather is, the better also.

I became attracted to and began to foster an internal theme of 'mental toughness'. I remember reading a book my girlfriend suggested on mental toughness training. I adopted a 'grin and bear it' attitude. I will do whatever it takes to get through those feelings and survive. No, strike that thought, I wanted to thrive! I also wanted badly to feel better during the year-end holidays.

One day a few years later, while I was in my mid-to-late thirties and now married to the girlfriend referred to earlier; it was thoughtfully brought to my attention that the use of light boxes was a way to combat Seasonal Affective Disorder, which I now prefer to characterize as 'light-deprivation'. What I read impressed me enough to cut it out and store it along with other items of particularly dubious value, in my junk drawer of course. ☺

Fast forward now to 1999 and lo and behold, I'm now divorced. During one especially dreary January, I became desperate. In that desperation, I began to rummage around and retrieved that article out from the drawer and read it again, this time with a particularly renewed intensity. Things hadn't exactly been all roses in my personal life for quite a while. I thank the good Lord for Duca, my then, faithful pet and companion Lakeland terrier, for being such a whimsical influence during these trying times.

And while we're at it, thank God for the Internet! Sorry Al Gore…you won't get credit for inventing the Internet from me, but I will mention you in passing because I believe you are generally a sincere man. (I saw somewhere that Al Gore is an Iron Maiden fan. I don't know if I believe it.)

Anyhow, after some lengthy searching, there was no Google then and things took real time to research, I picked up the phone and urgently placed an order for a light box and had it shipped PRIORITY. It arrived several days later. My Dad was visiting me when it arrived. I'm sure he was very confused and wondered what was causing this grown son of his to appear to be in such dire need.

But very much like a child that had simply opened the best Christmas present ever, I unpacked it and proudly placed it on my home workstation where it has remained since (at least during late fall, early winter, and any long stretches of rainy, cloudy weather.)

I confess. I'm not an expert in the clinical diagnosis of SAD. Nor do I know the specific biochemical or physiological basis for how SAD manifests itself in the human body. Most folks you encounter in the healthcare business don't understand it to that level of depth either. They're making tremendous progress and I'm sure that someday they'll have this all figured out. Until then, I reason it to myself in the following way. When people are healed by psychotherapy, no one cares or bothers to ask how it all came about. With 'light-deprivation induced mood attenuation' or 'LDIMA', which happens to be my abbreviation or buzzword of preference, no one will really care either. Relief is what matters most.

In fact, from here on in, when I'm referring to 'SAD', I'm going to give myself free reign to substitute 'LDIMA', because I think it gets right to the heart of the matter without having to tie it into a particular 'season' or make references to anything resembling a 'disorder'. It's entirely within the natural order of things to expect that human beings, whose ancestors evolved under the influence of the sun, feel ill at ease when deprived of that which helped bring about who they are today. The word 'Affective' is simply plain nonsense and was probably thrown in to make a word that resembled the mood of the people who were 'affected', as it were. You're not 'affected' when you have LDIMA, you are 'deprived'. The sooner you reorient yourself to this metaphor, the quicker you'll come to see things in the proper perspective. This perspective empowers you to take responsibility for your situation and there's plenty you can do about it.

No physician has ever formally diagnosed me. But please allow me to tell you this. It isn't necessary to seek a formal diagnosis to determine whether you have it, nor to resolve its symptoms. If I can do it, you can do it too.

You need not suffer the embarrassment of searching for answers from people who haven't experienced this for themselves. Read this short book, get out on the internet and do some research. You will learn what you need to know to overcome this on your own terms and with little, if any, medical intervention.

I don't mean to imply that you must avoid getting a medical diagnosis. If you are the type that relishes in knowing in detail, the minutiae of medical conditions, then please have at it. You'll simply have to get that somewhere else, meaning of course, not in this book. But please try my website, http://www.ldima.com. I keep a feed of the latest articles on SAD there along with other useful and some possibly useless, but whimsical news articles. I'll leave that for you to determine. As for myself, I simply got to the point where I wanted 'it' to be over. That is, I wanted to no longer be affected by light-deprivation.

On a more serious note, if you ever experience suicidal feelings, you are probably not susceptible to LDIMA but instead, have some form of depression entirely coincidental with winter and I strongly urge you to seek professional help immediately. There are links to a checklist on the Light of Day website of severe depressive symptoms.

It's 'sad', (pun intended this time) to say, but, SAD is not well understood by some primary care physicians and their counterparts in the nursing profession. I don't fault them, it's confusing. But we've also come a long way and public awareness has grown tremendously. How much attention do you expect to receive from the medical community for something that tends to resolve itself naturally if given enough time? This is one health issue that is well suited for attention from the self-help community.

What this book does not address is the so-called 'Summer SAD'.

Summer SAD is when you get depressed because of excessive exposure to daylight (and heat?) It doesn't seem reasonable that it would have anything to do with LDIMA, that's for sure. This does not happen to me either, I love heat and humidity.

I didn't find this regimen on the Internet; it grew out of my natural curiosity and from trial and error. I did read some books. I was able to take the best of my experiences and learn from others what was not working particularly well for them.

LDIMA symptoms are sometimes misconstrued as those normally attributed to depression. With even the best of intentions, your experience may have come to resemble mine. You may have found your doctor or nurse practitioner has given you a very limited and resoundingly inadequate treatment program. Worse still, you may be diagnosed as having a form of depression instead of being susceptible to light-deprivation and placed on harmful anti-depressant medications such as Zoloft. I know. I've been there too. See the article in the Appendix that appeared on the Internet during January of 2007 to see what I consider misinformation that is regularly handed out by professionals in the community in an attempt to educate the public. Take whatever side you wish, I believe in a more empowering paradigm, one where you have more control, with freedom from labels and shame.

Currently there is a growing buzz over either isolating or combining blue light in light therapy. I'm in the process of setting myself up to use a combination blue/white light therapy box for the coming season; I'll let you know how this goes. By the way, I'm always on the lookout for the 'FAD' in SAD treatment. This book will concentrate on a subset of self-proven treatment that will have you feeling your best. I've heard it said that 'luck is the residue of good design'. In this program, please consider the hypnosis as 'luck'. It may become the residue that remains in your life once the light therapy has terminated.

It isn't necessary to suffer the embarrassment of involving the medical and benefits departments of your workplace as you seek relief, or to be the brunt of jokes or strange looks from friends or well-intentioned co-workers who wonder what happened to the person who used to smile more often. Do check to see if you can be reimbursed for the light box.

Still, things are ever so slowly changing. With the advances these days it's possible to replace your task lamp at work with a fashionable 10,000-lux capable light therapy device. I simply don't recommend it, unless you have a plant that doesn't do too well in the off-season. ☺ I am a strong believer in home-administered light therapy and hypnosis.

The biggest of all the breakthroughs came when I finally realized how much negative thinking I had allowed to penetrate and reside in my unconscious. Many years ago, while I was a consultant working at Merrill Lynch, I had a friend who nicknamed me both 'super-Larry' and 'minus-Larry', depending upon what time of the year it was.

I never gave it much thought until one day many years later. I was driving to Guitar Center in Buffalo to get some new strings and to show off to my father a guitar similar to one I had recently purchased. I was looking to park the car when my Dad turned to me and said, "I don't know why you're bothering, you'll never learn to play that thing".

The light bulb went on 'big-time' in my head. I was staring at the person (not all that lovingly either, although I really do cherish my father) who no doubt once served as the 'ground-zero' for a measure of the negative thinking in my life. I didn't realize it right away, after all, that's my style if you haven't noticed already. But that experience did not recede into the backwaters of my mind and instead began to fester in my consciousness.

I slowly began to notice who was a positive force in my life and who was negative. I also began to search for something to help drive out the negativity that seemed to inhabit me. It was everywhere I looked and I have a dirty little secret to share. It still is everywhere, simply not in me so much anymore.

Shortly after that, I noticed that DirecTV had added XM radio to the lineup of channels I received as part of my monthly package. Being naturally curious, I flipped through them one day and got hung up on 'The System', the channel that presents 'electronic dance music in a relentless and uncompromising manner'. They're not kidding either! I began to listen whenever I was home or simply puttering around the house. It really lifted my level of motivation.

It eventually dawned on me one day while I was lost in thought that perhaps there was something more to this 'trance' music. I was noticing how I felt more positive while it played. It was only a short leap to go from the 'trance' in 'trance music' to the thought of considering using actual 'trance' to heal my negativity once and for all. From there it was only a few searches on Amazon.com before I found a hypnosis recording to help with self-confidence and self-esteem. If light therapy formed the foundation of my protocol, then the perfect accompaniment in hypnosis had finally been discovered.

I couldn't wait to try this. It wasn't even fall yet either. How amazing, another June-like miracle!

My solution does not involve the use of prescription medicine. You may need a prescription to obtain vitamin D in a dosage required for convenience sake. I do recommend involving your physician if you are already in treatment for depression or some other mood disorder. By all means, if you are currently taking an anti-depressant, read about and seriously consider substituting Saint John's Wort, if at all possible. The relative lack of side effects is a blessing. Warning: your mileage may vary.

Most people underestimate how important lifestyle adaptation is to coping with LDIMA. Once you experience these changes for yourself, you may choose to make them a permanent part of your life, as I have. You may also develop a certain fondness for a genre of music considered noise by many. I used to be one of them too. Whether you do or not, please understand how strongly I feel about the manner in which I respond to this debilitating, somewhat seasonal and completely correctable condition. When I make references to certain parts of the year, simply shift the calendar by 6 months if you reside in the southern hemisphere?

I have spent a significant part of my life coming to terms with my periodic, mislabeled, so-called depressions and subsequent sparkling recoveries. I sincerely wish to share what I've learned. You will literally turn your life around in days!

No one knows for sure how many people are really affected by light-deprivation. I've read estimates ranging from 2% of the population of the US to 10% of population of Canada. I think it's higher. I think it affects nearly everyone to some degree with the 2-10% numbers reserved for only the most seriously deprived. Ask spring-breakers, those kids go nuts when they get down south after being cooped up north all winter.

So, you think you have Seasonal Affective Disorder, do you? Do you want a way to find out for sure? Are you sick and tired of felling sick and tired? Are you ready to resolve this riddle once and for all by taking powerful and positive action? I know you are, after all, that's why you're here in the first place. But first, let's discuss LDIMA and how one behaves in May & June…

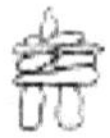

EFFORTLESS LIVING, LAZY & LONG DAYS

"I 'cloud nine' when I want too..."
Sly & the Family Stone – Hot Fun in the Summertime

SAD is categorized in DSM-IV as a form of bipolar mental disorder, manic in summer, depressed in winter.

Whatever...

I don't know about you, but I would definitely resent that label if someone were to actually tell me that was what SAD was. The last thing you need when you're dealing with light-deprivation is to have someone hang that one on you for size. It's disgusting.

I recently had the pleasure of meeting the physician and best-selling author Dr. John E. Sarno. It was pleasurable for me, not for the patient I so gingerly shepherded to his office at NYU, who was nearly completely incapacitated by lower back pain.

In Dr. Sarno's book, The Mindbody Prescription, he makes the case and it's a good one, that DSM fails to recognize psychosomatic disorders. They don't do much for the LDIMA patient either. Calling LDIMA a bipolar disorder may satisfy the 'category'-istas in this world, but it really does nothing more than drag down the self-esteem of the light-deprived person. I suggest that after you've read the above, you put it out of your mind, forever.

I wish I hadn't written it actually. But there it is. I actually went over this text quite a few times to replace 'depression' with 'light-deprivation' because I do not want you to think that I, even for a second, equate the two. They aren't. It is so easy to remediate light-deprivation and not so easy for the other. This is where I part company with those in the medical profession who prefer to place you on a less than natural regimen of pharmaceuticals; when a good dose of light, the carefully spoken word, a little dance music and some herbal-based supplements will bring relief with few side-effects.

During my first and really only serious attempt at obtaining a medical diagnosis, I contacted a physician who was involved with a sleep disorder clinic in New York City. At that time, I was taking St. John's Wort to combat what I then considered to be post-traumatic anxiety as a result of my then-recent divorce. I was beginning light therapy and part of the commitment I needed to make to gain admission into the sleep disorder program was to eliminate everything that I was currently doing and taking to then notice how well I did or did not sleep.

That was really too much to ask.

After dwelling on the options before me, I chose to not participate in the sleep disorder program. I'm so glad I followed my intuition. I couldn't imagine what the benefit was to me of discontinuing the noticeable relief I was experiencing, only to put myself through what was certain to be a return to the uncomfortable conditions I had left behind, in the hopes of coming closer to a diagnosis. There had to be another way. This is why I now refuse to take recommendations from anyone who hasn't already 'walked a mile in my shoes' or something similar to it.

I'm not sure how SAD came to fall within this categorization in DSM. But I do understand the difference in how I have felt nearer the summer as compared to the winter solstice. Part of what makes LDIMA so unsettling is the long, steady attenuation in mood that occurs in the light deprived as the days dwindle down towards the end of the year. I used to consider this 'normal'. If you think this happens to you, please take note.

'Attenuation' is typically defined as the reduction in strength of a signal. I consider 'mood attenuation' to be the reduction in intensity of positive feelings as the amount of available light decreases.

Equally amazing and a tribute to the ability of the human body is the recovery that spontaneously occurs as the days lengthen after New Years, culminating in the effortless feeling that those with LDIMA enjoy as the beginning of summer approaches.

To me, there's nothing more enjoyable than lying out on the back deck in late May and early June, before the summers heat and humidity arrive. Listening to the birds chirp and watching the sky slowly darken as the stars begin to appear, the lazy long days of late spring and early summer bring unparalleled feelings of serenity and contentment. It's like a naturally euphoric drug.

Long periods of daylight bring out the very best in mood for the light deprived. You may even entertain the thought that what felt so lousy last winter was merely a figment of your imagination. Everything seems so effortless in June.

Now, let's return to where we were earlier. Perhaps it is now, but if not, then imagine it's late fall. That's the perfect time to learn whether you truly are light deprived and for this we need to plan a getaway.

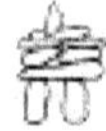

DESTINATION: HEAD SOUTH, REALLY FAR SOUTH

"Let the sun shine, let the sunshine in, the sunshine in..."
The Fifth Dimension - Acquarius/Let The Sunshine In

Location: Somewhere far south

Agenda: Book a mini-vacation in sunny, southern Florida for late December. December 19-23 is be the perfect time; although anytime from late November to early January will be equally as sufficient. The first week of December is traditionally a slow travel time and you may be able to find a bargain then.

While you are there, get active again! Go in the hot tub first thing every morning for a morning soak. Swim in the pool each and every day, if they don't have one, swim in the ocean. Rent a bicycle and ride the beach. Drench yourself in the available light of day.

Visit local parks and go bird watching, eat summer-like salads and drink plenty of water. Remember to apply your sunscreen liberally. If you are already taking SJW, try an alternative schedule where you delay all but the morning dose until the strong light of day has passed. During my visits to test this therapy I refrained from taking SJW after my breakfast dose until after 5 PM and then take the remaining doses in a spread out fashion over the hours left before retiring for the night.

Watch the sunset every evening and go for walks on the beach at night. While you're out on the beach at night, look up at all the stars! This is what you've been missing!! This is what your body needs to feel whole again.

Four to five days will be enough to reset your body in preparation for what will certainly reassert itself upon your return if LDIMA is what is truly affecting you. Mark your calendar now and remember to follow through. You'll be glad you did, for this is how I diagnosed myself.

Now, here's another little telltale sign that you may have LDIMA. Do you experience feelings of desperation the closer you get to the winter solstice? If you find yourself frantically making purchases to try to alleviate these feelings, say, by self-educating yourself in some promising alternative therapy, like yoga, meditation or perhaps sun-gazing? Sun gazing sounds like exactly what the SAD doctor would order for himself, doesn't it? The chances are good these feelings of urgency and desperation are simply another LDIMA symptom, a companion to the dread. Maybe you eat more or drink alcohol instead?

By all means, buy the book or tape or whatever it is you, in desperation, feel drawn to. It's a good time of the year to have a learning agenda. I highly recommend it. But be prepared to resell whatever you've purchased next spring on Amazon.com as you will probably look back and wonder why you were so sure you had to make that purchase in the first place. I'm often exactly like this and it's really funny to watch it happen to me even when I know better!

Here's a tip that will help recoup more than what you paid for this book and then some. Use the website Amazon.com to sell some of the more valuable stuff you've been accumulating in your home over the years! I've made thousands of dollars unloading my old books. Others will be glad you did this too! It's something else you will do while you're sitting in front of the light-box; you will post your books for sale online and manage your sales account. Please keep this book though! I'd be happy to autograph it so that it has 'collectible' status. ☺

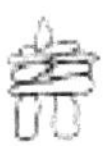

UPON RETURNING FROM YOUR VACATION

"Oh the wind can carry, I'll stand in the light"
Rush - Available Light

I'm a huge fan of the Canadian band Rush. The lyrics above close out the song 'Available Light' on the 'Presto' recording.

Neil Peart, the drummer of Rush, writes the lyrics for the band and those who know me well also know I haven't been the same since the summer of 2002. I was traveling in California and during a site tour given by the folks from one of the companies I am affilated with, I was graciously offered 10th row tickets and valet parking to spend an evening at a Rush concert at the Shoreline Amphitheatre.

As you now know, I grew up in western New York and Rush was very popular and always touring in the late 70's and early 80's and despite this alleged availability, I neglected to see them even though I had been offered a similar set of tickets right around the time of the Moving Pictures tour. Looking back, I really regret not getting to see them earlier. But I digress.

At the time I was in California, I had also been reading Neil's book, Ghost Rider. It's an accounting of a motorcycle trip Neil made after the tragic deaths of both his daughter and the some months later, his wife.

Neil alludes to having Seasonal Affective Disorder during the part of the book where he's holed up in his home in Quebec. I always wondered why his lyrics resonated so well with me and I'm not sure, but I have this theory that it has to do with LDIMA somehow. Rush is really popular in Canada and understandably so as they're a genuine Canadian band. I grew up 8 miles from Canada and I sometimes feel very Canadian, especially when watching hockey. While I lack the vernacular and pronunciation style of the nearby residents of the province of Ontario, I certainly enjoy traveling in Canada and try to slip across the border whenever I'm visiting my family.

I have this baseless theory that there are a lot of people who have LDIMA in Canada and like myself, we somehow have this affection for rock music that is at least partly LDIMA inspired. Anyway, the Shoreline concert was magnificent. I only recognized one song, the opener; but I loved everything I heard that night. It was a truly magical evening for me.

Ok, you've taken your vacation and returned. I hope you remembered to take your sunscreen to help cushion the shock your body will receive when it experiences the drastic difference in sunlight intensity. If you're like me you'll feel really great for a day or two but after a week or so you'll have slipped back into feeling that dreadful feeling that something is missing, especially if you aren't doing anything about your light-deprivation. It's not your imagination either. What's missing is the quality and strength of light necessary for optimal living. You are not getting your minimum daily requirement of light.

While away, you may have also noticed a pleasant up-tick in your sex drive that occurred while you were getting more light exposure. If that happened for you, then congratulations!

You're definitely a valid candidate and certainly ready for this therapy. You may be even if this didn't happen for you depending on other factors in your life.

To prepare, acquire at least the first two of the following items:

1) **A minimum 10,000-lux full-spectrum light box,** preferably one that does not emit ultra-violet light rays. I use an Ott bioLIGHTSYSTEMS™ WinterBright 2001Biolight. This is not an endorsement, use whatever fits your taste and budget.

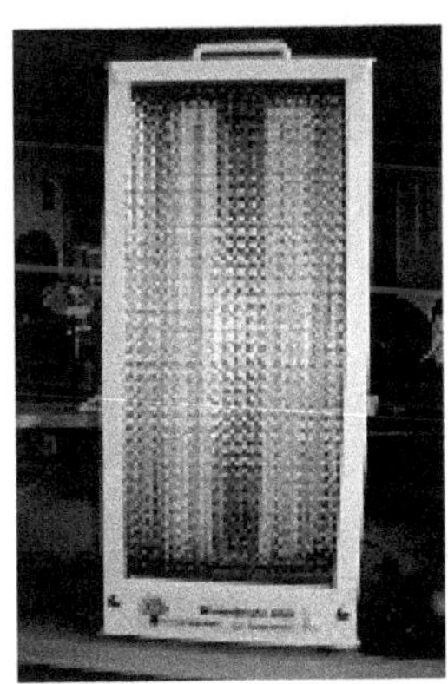

Please avoid a box that emits UV radiation. Buy as much light box as your budget will allow, the bigger, more expensive boxes may be used from a greater distance and will literally drench you in beneficial, healing light.

You may want to purchase or borrow a light meter to help find the optimum distance for receiving a 10,000-lux dose and to help determining the boundaries for proper positioning. It is necessary for me to sit with my nose level with the middle of the light box and no further from the light box than the distance from the tip of my thumb to the tip of my pinky finger with my fingers spread wide, about 9 ½ inches. This is pretty close!

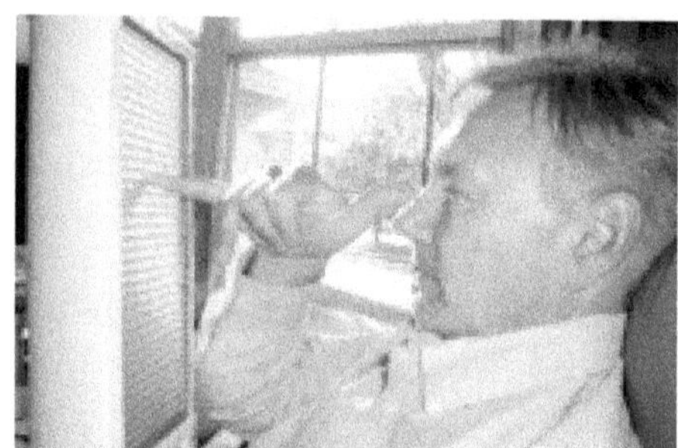

I verified that I am receiving a 10,000 lux dose at that distance with an LX1010B light meter shown here.

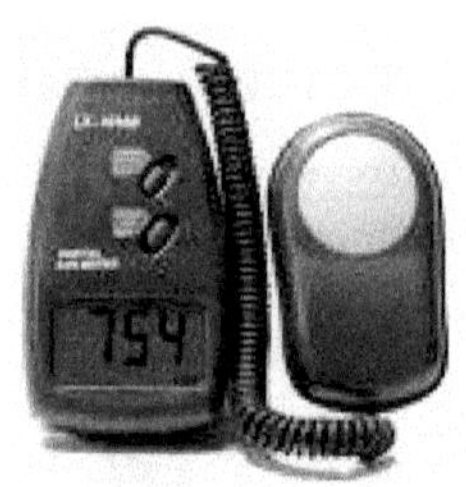

There is no brand name on the meter I used. It's from China and its purpose was to measure light for orchids. You may be able to find something like it on the Internet or at your local garden center. What I like about the meter is that it has three thresholds for measurement. One for very low light conditions, under 2,000 lux. One for medium light conditions of 2,000 to 50,000 lux and one for above 50,000 lux.

While we're on the subject, I measured the light received under various conditions to see how deficient or well lit some of the areas I frequently spend time in may be. It was an effort I made to try to determine a minimum daily requirement of light for myself, which I still haven't accurately determined, but believe to be important to have an idea about.

What do you think is the amount of light registered on the light meter in each of the following scenarios? Each measurement is taken from eye level during the month of January.

1. Standing at the sink of my interior bathroom (no windows), lit with eight 40-watt bulbs in a mirrored strip light. The dimmer is set to full on. (Answer: 325 lux)
2. Standing at night, near the center of a 13' x 18' bedroom, 2 lamps lit with 50-200-250 watt 3-way light bulbs (on the middle setting, 200 watts) placed on nightstands on both sides of the bed along with 1 75- watt light bulb in a third pinup lamp across the room placed on a console styled television? (Answer: ~67 lux)
3. Standing outside at 9 AM, cloudless sky, facing the sun, which is shining brightly in mid-January in New Brunswick, NJ? (Answer 90,000+ lux)
4. Sitting in front of a double-hung window at my workstation at home, 8 AM, it's cloudy. There are trees with no leaves obstructing some of the sky.
(Answer: 190 lux)

That's quite a bit of variability and it helps to explain why the relative lack of light in winter results in LDIMA for those affected. It becomes difficult to obtain your minimum daily requirement of light, especially if you can't get outside.

2) **A hypnosis recording for the enhancement of self-esteem.** While I was developing my program I was using a recording by Janet Decker for self-confidence and self-esteem (use whatever you prefer.) I picked the recording I did because it used specific phrasing about "seeing yourself in a 'light' that is totally different" and as a certified hypnotist, I have come to know that good hypnotherapy is metaphorically superior.

3) **A 'trance' music recording** (this is optional). Please see a physician if you have any heart-related concerns. All we're trying to do here is jump-start or extend the elevation of mood by increasing your heartbeat while indoors. That way, you won't have to exercise outside if the weather is horrendous. I'm aware that many readers may live where it is very cold, like my former home at the 'North Pole', e.g., Buffalo, NY. ☺ It's also a good pick-me-up for listening in the car as you travel about, regardless of the time of year.

4) **A 90-day supply of St. John's Wort** (again, optional). 90 days may not be enough to last the full season but it's a start. You may use some of the online tools I present in

the Appendix to determine how long to expect to be in light therapy and then purchase accordingly.

5) **Vitamin D, 50,000 iu dosage** (optional, please know you may need a prescription for this and should have your blood tested to make sure you need supplementation, if you do, ask for 24), that's more than enough if you take one a week.

Before we continue, let's take a moment to rethink one item…

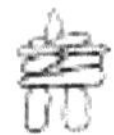

REDEFINING A 'DAY'

"I believe in what I see
I believe in what I hear
I believe that what I'm feeling
Changes how the world appears"
Rush – 'Totem'

To really understand how your body will respond to this combination therapies, it is necessary to re-think the generally accepted definition of a 'day'. Most people think of a day as starting when they awake from sleep and ending when they return to bed, for that is the generally accepted way. For the purposes of this combination of strategies, a 'day' begins when you begin to prepare for sleep. Why is this?

I'd like to draw for you, an analogy to taking a trip, say on motorcycle. You don't simply jump on the bike and take off. Before leaving, you make sure the gas tank was full, that there was sufficient air in the tires and your possessions firmly secured. You want to make sure you had sufficient rest and that you were properly nourished as piloting a motorcycle requires your undivided attention.

So your trip really begins with the preparations you make the night before. This preparation continues immediately after you rise the next morning as you bathe, eat and then pack your possessions onto the motorcycle. You may think of the trip as already having begun as soon as you begin to prepare the night before. You've started the chain of events that need to occur to have a safe, successful outcome.

It's kind of the same thing with light therapy and hypnosis. In order to ensure that your 'work day' or whatever it is that you will be doing has the greatest chance of success, you need to begin to make preparations the night before and for the light deprived, even more so. Consistent sleep habits are of paramount importance to successfully overcoming LDIMA. Preparation for sleep is the key. This therapy relies heavily and obtains the majority of its benefit by sandwiching sleep between the highest quality of coincident light and hypnotherapeutic treatment. The hypnotic sessions will be conducted in front of a 10,000-lux minimum light box that emits full-spectrum light (minus that within the UV spectrum, if desired).

If you deem it necessary, regularly scheduled supplementation with Saint John's Wort will help to bring an additional elevation in mood and provide stability throughout the season. The author uses a brand of SJW that has been standardized to deliver a consistent dosage. Avoid the gel caps of the crushed herb, they do not age well and have been found to be inconsistent in formal testing conducted by respected authorities.

Choose a brand that is of pharmaceutical quality and easily available over-the-counter.

How do you decide if SJW supplementation is necessary? I found I needed an extra lift during the time when I was experiencing seasonal light-deprivation. I'm a firm believer in 'start wherever you are' and I believe in healing yourself in real-time, on the spot, whenever necessary. While strictly my personal experience, the content of my dreams will often contain a subtle threat of violence when I abstain from or withdraw SJW during periods of light-deprivation. You may have another way to tell, each person is different.

Another way I know is the way I feel in the morning after awakening. A heavy sensation on my upper cheekbones immediately beneath the skin surface coincidental with a lingering sensation of morning sluggishness is enough to convince me that I need to begin SJW supplementation and perhaps a longer light therapy session too.

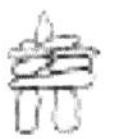

THE PROGRAM

"I want a new drug, one with no doubts, one that won't keep me up all night, or make my face breakout..."
Huey Lewis - ' I Want a New Drug'

To achieve the best result, each evening, before retiring to sleep and depending upon the recording you have selected, you will be spending approximately 25 to 30 minutes listening to the 'payload' selection of a self-esteem hypnosis recording. I use the term 'payload' because often, hypnosis recordings come with multiple tracks. One track may contain an abundance of positive suggestions and inferences (hence the term 'payload') with the other containing suggestions to promote deep relaxation only. You will do this facing the lighted light box. Feel free to rotate among several hypnotic recordings if you are fortunate or interested enough to have acquired more than one. As a beginner new to hypnosis and working for the first time to overcome LDIMA, you will not find a better recording to start with than 'Hypnosis for Self-Confidence and Self-Esteem' by Janet Decker.

Hypnosis benefits the light-deprived person by deeply planting many correlated positive suggestions and then allowing the unwanted negativity and its associated unresolved emotions, thoughts and feelings to 'vent' out later during the sleep that follows. This venting process occurs naturally during the third and last stage of sleep.

According to Dr. John Kappas, the body at sleep goes through three sleep stages. The first stage of your sleep contains 'wishful thinking' dreams and occurs during the first two hours of sleep. The middle stage contains what is known as 'precognitive' dreams. If you are ever awakened and have an 'aha' moment, it is occurring during the precognitive stage of sleep. The third and final phase is known as the 'venting' stage, where negative inputs are removed.

Your body will not simply divide whatever sleep-time you give it into thirds to accomplish its dream work, as it does not know in advance whether you will obtain the necessary length of rest. So if you do not give it nearly 8 hours of sleep each night, you will not get to the third stage of dreamtime needed for this venting process to occur. If a full nights rest is less than eight hours for you, that is perfectly okay. I tend to average a little over seven hours of sleep a night. Your experience may be different.

To repeat, to maximize your success, it is important to get a full nights rest each night while using this program. The more regular your sleep habits become, the more 'normal' you will come to feel upon rising the following morning. Fortunately, for many people susceptible to LDIMA, they tend to want to get a lot of sleep. But this is not the rule for all who are light deprived. Some of these susceptible individuals do not easily sleep well. Hypnosis will greatly benefit these folks by providing a regular period of progressive relaxation immediately prior to retiring to sleep.

Again, conduct your late evening hypnosis session with the light box on, eyes closed. I have not found light therapy in the late evening to interfere with the quality of my sleep or to inhibit the onset of drowsiness; the hypnosis takes care of that. If you find that this is not the case for you, do not use the light box and listen to the hypnosis recording only. Instead, try including a light-therapy session coincident with either track of your hypnosis recording earlier in the evening, perhaps upon returning home from work or after dinner.

Remember to keep the corners of your mouth turned up all the while as the hypnosis recording plays, that is, to 'smile'. Your brain has linked an abundance of positive feelings with smiling and smiling during hypnosis will help return the brain to a more positive place naturally. There have been studies that have concluded that 'smile' therapy alone can be helpful in lifting mood dramatically, if given enough time and repetition

Strive to breath deeply and diaphragmatically, especially during the initial phases of your hypnosis sessions as this helps to promote a deeper relaxation. Diaphragmatic breathing happens when you push your belly muscles out as you breathe in deeply, and then pull your belly muscles in as you expel the breath on exhalation.

Sleep is to commence shortly after finishing your late evening hypnosis. Here's a simple exercise to do immediately prior turning out the lights. Keep a journal next to your bed along with a pen. Write the following sentence in your journal longhand 10 times before going to sleep:

'I have overcome the effects of light-deprivation.'

Do this for a minimum of three weeks or at least until you no longer feel the pangs of light-deprivation, whichever takes longer. Trust your instincts to know when it is okay to discontinue the journaling. As with other parts of this program, resume the journaling whenever you begin to experience the subtle effects of light-deprivation again.

You may also wish to record whether the day has been a rewarding day or a challenging one. Simply write a capital 'R' or capital 'C' in your journal. Challenging isn't to be viewed in a negative light, as the challenge is well met when you make the next day a rewarding one. You will prepare yourself best for the day to come by following this program in a consistent fashion. After a while, count up your 'R's and 'C's. Over time, the frequency of 'C's will dwindle if not disappear entirely.

Why does this journaling help, you ask?

The beauty of writing in longhand is that what you will write shortly before going to sleep will be interpreted by the mind as a form of hypnotic suggestion. These writings bypass what is known as the 'critical area of mind' and are simply another form of self-hypnosis. If you have an objection to journaling, please know that it is perfectly acceptable to 'grind-in' this new expectation by reciting it aloud or to yourself silently, aloud is preferable.

In this book I make reference to two different forms of hypnosis, self-hypnosis and hetero-hypnosis. In actuality, most hypnosis is hetero-hypnosis. Hetero-hypnosis is any form of hypnosis in which you are not the 'director'. Using a recording such as you will in this program is a form of hetero-hypnosis and it succeeds by overwhelming the critical area of mind. When you use the services of a hypnotherapist, you are also submitting yourself to hetero-hypnosis, regardless of the gender of the hypnotherapist. In this case, 'hetero' means 'other than yourself'.

Self-hypnosis is a process by which you, on your own, organize your thought process and in this organization, succeed in bypassing this same critical area of mind, using a more direct and deliberate approach.

In a later chapter I will introduce you to a quick form of self-hypnosis I sometimes use to reinforce my personal agenda and to plant helpful suggestions. This has helped me tremendously, especially when I do not have time to set aside for a more thorough relaxation induction and hypnotic session, like that used in this therapy when listening to the hypnotic recording.

Immediately upon rising the next morning, you will repeat the 'payload' hypnosis session while seated in front of the light box with your eyes closed and the light box on. To repeat, the light box may be close to your face so that you get the maximum benefit through closed eyelids. The only thing I suggest to do after rising other than going to the bathroom is to take any supplements, if you are using them. Do not fall out of the habit of doing hypnosis with light therapy immediately upon rising. It's that important to the effort of artificially extending the perceived length of daylight and reinforcing a positive hypnotic agenda.

Remember to check with the manufacturer to find out what distance from the light box corresponds to a dose of 10,000 lux or measure it yourself if you have a light meter. Upon completing the hypnosis session, I turn off the light box immediately before opening my eyes. If you do not turn it off, it may momentarily dazzle you. It will help if you synchronize your session so that it concludes coincident with sunrise. This will also help to artificially lengthen the amount of time your body perceives as daytime.

I know I seem to be repeating myself, but your eyelids must always remain closed when using the light box, especially if you choose to supplement with St. John's Wort. SJW causes sensitivity of the skin and eyes to bright light, that's part of how it helps to alleviate the unwelcome effects of light-deprivation. My light box has never burned me, however I am concerned about my eyes. So please keep your eyes closed when using the light box. The light from a 10,000-lux light-box is plenty strong enough to penetrate the eyelids and deliver effective light-therapy when used in this way.

The widely accepted method of receiving light therapy is to have your eyes open but to not be looking directly into the light box. That is to allow the light to enter your eye without requiring you to stare directly at the light box. I have many reasons to support performing light therapy with the eyes closed, here are my top three:

1) I've tried it and it works equally as well as long as the dosage hitting the middle of your forehead is 10,000 lux or greater

2) Light reaches the pineal gland and begins its healthful remediation without traveling strictly through the open eyes; it does not need to enter solely through the retina either. There is evidence that the pineal gland receives stimulation through other avenues of the nervous system

3) If you've ever sat facing the sun in mid-winter, you soon realize how beneficial the sun shining on your face feels. It's overpoweringly wonderful and you do not need to experience it with eyes open, any sunbather will attest to this. On a clear day in mid-winter, light strength may register anywhere from 30,000 to in excess of 90,000 lux, depending upon the time of day and height of the sun in the sky. This is the absolutely best light therapy of all. Like the song says, "there's nothing like the real thing!"

My own experience has led me to conclude that always having your eyes closed is the safest way to go. The pineal gland is responsible for the production of melatonin and serotonin in the body and those with LDIMA must be over-producing melatonin and under-producing serotonin. I don't mean to imply that there is anything particularly wrong with the pineal glands of those with LDIMA either.

It's simply a case of the gland doing what it does naturally, depending of course on the amount and strength of available light. Exposure to light means the pineal gland will tend to curtail its melatonin production and instead increase serotonin production. I like to use light therapy immediately before I go to bed precisely because it interrupts the pineal glands natural melatonin producing cycle and provides the opportunity for a burst of serotonin immediately prior to the onset of sleep.

Authors Robert Becker and Gary Selden make the argument in the book, The Body Electric, that certain experiments concerning magnetism and its affect on circadian rhythms had to be controlled for light exposure as 'it has been known for several years that shining a light on the head somehow modifies the (*pineal*) gland's hormone output even though it's buried so deeply within the head in most vertebrates that, as far as we know, it can't react directly to the light'.

Okay, so enough about the eyes open vs. eyes shut already. Besides, the hypnosis recordings will all instruct you to close your eyes anyway! Follow the recording's advice and 'just do it'. ☺

You may feel your eyes move about under your eyelids as you respond to the hypnosis. This is common and normal. They may also want to roll up under your eyelids. Again, this is common and considered normal. If you feel as though you aren't actually entering a hypnotic trance, which some people believe, try gently rolling your eyeballs up under your eyelids to see if this enhances your ability to enter trance. Either way, no matter how much you resist, you will enter trance eventually.

I don't want to belabor how to, or whether you enter trance, but I would like to offer some additional background if you question whether you really enter a trance state. Please see the later chapter on hypnosis, it offers some helpful information. The important point is that everyone can experience hypnosis.

At this point you have the tools necessary to remediate light deprivation. What follows is something that I offer as additional modalities designed to complement the work you will do above. They are by no means a required activity but I have found them to be effective during the very darkest times of the year, around the solstice.

After you have completed the combined hypnosis and light therapy, if it moves you to do so, begin listening to some trance music as you prepare for work or continue your morning routine. Your heart will sync up with the beat of the music (approximately 140 beats per minute) by a process known as 'entrainment' and this will propel you forward through the early part of the morning with increased vigor.

Now, I realize that not everyone is going to take to 'trance' music. It tends to be more attractive to a younger mindset. The dance crowd comes to mind initially. You will accomplish pretty much the same thing without trance music by using a metronome. An inexpensive Korg unit will run for under $30 and it can be set up to beat at a wide range. Use 140-148 beats per minute (BPM) to simulate the affect you receive from trance music. Try to find something that will beat loudly. I like trance music because the beat will often be felt throughout the house.

While in the car on the way to work, I often listen to audio books that I call my 'success coach' recordings. These continue the process of installing additional positive and motivating messages, which are so important at this potentially fragile time of the year. I avoid listening to the news, any potentially uninspiring music or broadcast commentary from Thanksgiving through the end of January. It's nice to take a break from the news. The famed integrative medicine physician, Dr. Andrew Weil, has suggested this to be good for anyone to do periodically. Why not start today? I find that when I've returned to listening to the news, that I haven't missed anything. In its place, I gain an increased appreciation for and focus on my own personal agenda. The concentration has a powerful and positive affect.

As mentioned briefly before, upon returning from work or shortly after the sun sets, if you do not leave the house during the day, it is often helpful to have another light therapy session with hypnosis.

For this session, you may choose to use the relaxation track on the recording, if one has been provided, while you repeat the light therapy. If you are using the Decker recording previously suggested, this session will last about 20 minutes and again will help to extend the length of time your body perceives as daylight. If you fall asleep, the extra light will do you no harm.

The relaxation sessions will also do wonders for anything else on your plate', whether it be hypertension, periodic stress and tension, or anger. Who among us will not benefit from a little extra relaxation, especially after a long day at work or stressful commute home?

It's also quite likely that on some days you may feel more in need of light, particularly if there have been a number of cloudy days in a row, which may happen at any time of the year. Don't be bashful about extending the light and hypnosis sessions. The nice thing about many hypnosis recordings is that they often contain two hypnosis sessions that may be listened to back-to-back along with light therapy, extending your 25-minute sessions out to 45 minutes or longer. Trust your body to tell you when you are in need of light and then give it what it craves. Over time, you will become the expert. This is knowledge of the highest order.

Finally, if you find after a blood test that you have become depleted, take the 50,000 IU of Vitamin D once a week to ensure you're getting adequate supplementation for what the sun ordinarily helps produce in the body. Start when you begin light therapy and eliminate it when you terminate light therapy.

You may always obtain a mid-season blood test to determine whether your levels of Vitamin D are adequate at this dosage or if you may need to make adjustments.

Should you desire additional light therapy, perhaps because you are new to the protocol, have recently acquired the equipment and want to get a really good dose, but feel that you need to do other things like reading or watching TV, try the following:

Place the light box on the floor so that it shines upwards onto the underside of your knees. You'll need to wear shorts to expose the backsides of your knees. Because it's likely to be winter, you may get chilly. Put a blanket on your lap and cover your legs. This will also prevent the light box from dazzling anyone who may be in the room with you. I found this very effective early in the season and will soon get by simply using only the morning and late-evening treatments.

I will now mention an alternative to light-box therapy that I'm considering trying one of these years and may become an addendum to this therapy once I have given it a go. I've always wanted to take a tanning canopy and replace the tanning bulbs with full-spectrum equivalents (minus UV rays) and lay underneath that in shorts instead of sitting in front of the light box.

I once read about a physician who created a similar device she called a light-bed and allowed her patients to use it when they were at her office. They loved it.

Another alternative is to use the natural supplementation that strong daylight allows. I do this on weekends when I am unable to sit outdoors, but you may adapt it to your 'light-style' as the opportunity allows. I lie on my bed propped up by pillows and face the bedroom window and allow the strong morning sunlight to shine on my face (eyes-closed) and if it is warm enough, I will roll up my sleeves and expose my arms to have more skin surface area exposed. I will listen to both tracks on the hypnosis CD back-to-back. This provides the most powerful boost of all the strategies in mid-winter. The sunlight coming in my window is typically above 30,000 lux and because the light passes through glass there is little to no UV danger. Do this; I believe you will love it! I think I know why my dog liked to sit in the bright sunlight as much as she did.

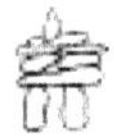

BEDROOM SETUP

"Now it's dark and I'm alone
but I won't be afraid
in my room"
The Beach Boys – 'In My Room'

In the ideal world of the light-deprived person, they have access to a bedroom with white or light-colored walls and ceilings, having a window facing east with an unobstructed view to the horizon. This allows the first light of day to enter the room with little if any degradation.

As luck has it, my bedroom faces east, but has some trees and another building obstructing my view of the horizon. It's also on the ground floor, the second floor would have been better, third floor better still. It is optimal to have no shades obstructing the view from your window, but not everyone feels comfortable with that arrangement.

So, if you were going to obstruct your window, it is beneficial to use the minimum opacity necessary for privacy. I use a bright white 1" opaque fabric mini-shade with no curtain. I have a valance to hide the blind hardware and no side curtains. I want as much natural light to enter the room ASAP in the morning. I leave the blinds down overnight and I raise them on sunny weekends, shortly after sunrise. Because my headboard backs up to the window, I am able to get the first light of the day shining onto my forehead. Having no headboard would be better. On sunny winter weekends, I reorient my position in bed after waking so that my feet are closest to the window instead of my head. I am able to allow the morning sun (if cloudless) to shine through the window and onto my face and body. Sometimes, I do the morning hypnosis session in this manner, when I'm not rising at or before dawn. (Yes, even I find it impossible to keep strictly to my own program, so there, I said it).

I have three lamps in my bedroom. On either nightstand you'll find a lamp that accommodates a three-way bulb. The bulbs I use are 50-200-250. Guess which setting I keep the lamps on at night? Of course, it's the 250-watt setting.

The third lamp sits atop my television and is a pinup lamp with a 75-watt clear bulb. I prefer clear or frosted bulbs. I tried the full spectrum bulbs and oddly, they had a 'creepy' feel to them. Normal incandescent lighting is 'warm' enough for my taste, so I recommend them. I don't care for the current types of compact fluorescent. Your mileage may very of course. I use the television in the bedroom more for the XM music stations than for TV itself.

I have an adjoining bathroom and it's lit by an eight-bulb mirrored strip light that is fully dimmable. Needless to say, when it's on, it's on full. I keep eight 40-watt bulbs in that fixture. I suggest you brighten the bathroom you use in the morning to the maximum.

Upon rising, I always turn the lights on full in the bedroom. I will take my supplements and immediately begin my morning light therapy and hypnosis session. I open the curtains to let as much light in as possible after I've finished bathing and have dressed, providing the sun has already risen.

Curiously, I don't use a dawn simulator. I may if I were unable to adjust my waking routine so that I am able to complete my morning light therapy at daybreak. One feature that I know would be helpful with a dawn simulator if it existed would be for it to know where it is in the time zone, like having a built-in Global Positioning System, so that it more accurately adjusts the brightening to artificially extend the day as much as possible without reprogramming as

GPS systems know the day of the year, time of sunrise and sunset. The integrated lamp simulators I've looked into do not allow much more than a 60-watt bulb to be used. I like things much brighter.

I tested the amount of available light coming through the white opaque shade of my bedroom window at dawn, it was a whopping 1-lux. Still, it was enough to arouse me from slumber. Your mileage may vary.

If I designed the ultimate dawn simulator, what will it look like? Here's a description. I would install a fluorescent fixture into the recess of my double-hung bedroom window so that it was hidden behind the valance (my drapery of choice)

and in front of the window shade. I would then swap out the existing tube, if one were included, for a full-spectrum bulb (full-spectrum fluorescent bulbs do not have that 'creepy' feel the incandescent have.) This fixture would be plugged into a dedicated dawn simulator device that occupies some available space on one of the nightstands.

I would obtain a simulator that does not have a light-bulb built-in, but instead has timing capabilities. Then, I'd program the fluorescent light to begin brightening roughly 30-45 minutes before my planned time to arise. This approximates a natural sunrise and the light will be originating roughly from the same location.

One thing you'll notice about this program is that I tend to err on the side of strength. I like to use brighter lighting, but I arrange it so that I am doing it safely. I like 50,000 IU of vitamin D weekly, not three 400 IU vitamin D soft gels daily. I have my blood tested periodically to be sure I'm not doing any harm.

As far as light therapy goes, I like to know where the sweet spot is for a minimum 10,000-lux session. I'll sometimes bring the light even closer, well made light therapy devices have the proper shielding built in, so it isn't going to harm you, but please be safe, keep your eyes closed.

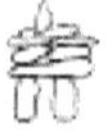

NO TIME FOR DEPRESSANTS

"Get up, get up, put your body in motion..."
Wiseguys - 'Start the Commotion'

Late fall and early winter are absolutely the worst time for anyone with LDIMA to even consider taking depressants. Please, do not drink alcohol or take sleeping aids. These are true 'external solutions'. They will leave you feeling worse in the morning, require more time to recover and reduce the effectiveness of the combined light & hypnosis therapies. If you drink, you'll soon find yourself backsliding and it is not very pleasant at all.

If you feel you simply must drink to be social, then plan to spend additional time in front the light box, perhaps while sobering up!

Alcohol combined with coffee or caffeine-rich soft drinks combined with alcohol are also not a good option, eventually, the caffeine is broken down in your body and you will be left with the residuals effects of the alcohol metabolism.

Now, any discussion of depressants or depressants mixed with stimulants will not be complete if we do not at least pay some lip service to pure stimulants alone. I've found that it is possible to substitute 'trance' music for coffee or tea in the morning or at any time of the day for that matter. This is a more natural way to raise the heart beat and has no residual effects such as the feeling of 'crashing' that caffeine addicts experience once the caffeine has been metabolized by the body. So, please try 'trance' music or any music with a consistent beat to it of at or around 140 beats per minute.

You have to find a way to continue or resume physical activity while in late-fall and early to mid-winter. Motion is the 'potion' and light fuels good feelings. Perhaps that means walking for an hour instead of riding your bicycle, or using a treadmill or stationary bicycle indoors while doing light therapy. Do whatever it takes to restore your level of in-season activity while off-season.

Another way to measure your level of activity is to wear a pedometer. These handy little step counters will help you to record your progress toward greater motion. Document your physical activity in your journal along with the light sessions and assessment of the level of your mood. Later on, you can look back to see what combination(s) provide the most benefit. 10,000 steps each day is a good goal for optimum health.

You may also want to investigate the Mental Bank Concept created by the noted author and hypnotherapist, Dr. John Kappas. The Mental Bank program describes a way of obtaining measurable improvements in finances, health, relationships; almost anything, by identifying 'value events' that have a previously assigned but artificial dollar value associated with them, depending upon your personal values, as well as the perceived importance or difficulty you assign to completing them. By recording these 'deposits' into a Mental Bank Account, you encourage yourself to do what you need to do to obtain these life improvements. I have a link to free streaming video provided by the Hypnosis Motivation Institute website in the appendix if you think this may be of interest to you.

I also recommend carrying a small voice recorder to temporarily store items to journal later in the day. You may also use it to store 'highly valued' thoughts that you may wish to repeat to yourself or action items to take in business or personal relationships.

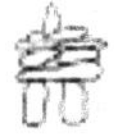

THE 'LIST'

"Some are blessed and some are cursed,
the golden one or scarred from birth,
while others only see the worst,
such a lot of pain on the earth"
Rush – 'The Larger Bowl'

If you've spent any amount of time researching SAD on the Internet, there's little doubt that you've come across websites that contain a list of symptoms associated with SAD. I've taken a sample of these symptoms from a site that will remain anonymous and reprinted them below.

- Depression with a fall or winter onset
- Lack of energy
- Decreased interest in work or significant activities
- Increased appetite with weight gain
- **Carbohydrate cravings**
- Increased sleep, excessive daytime sleepiness
- Social withdrawal

- Afternoon slumps with decreased energy and concentration
- Slow, sluggish, lethargic movement

After reading a list like this you may be tempted to agree that you indeed have some or perhaps all of the symptoms to some degree or another. I've found that dwelling on the symptoms, while initially helpful in trying to self-diagnose, is essentially a self-sabotaging endeavor in the long run as the time you spend in subsequent re-examination is much better spent on remediation.

Still, while the symptoms as presented above do some justice to the feelings that may accompany the light-deprived during periods of seasonal light variation or temporary deprivation, at least one of them is completely without merit and it concerns cravings.

The generally accepted opinion among SAD experts is that people will tend to crave carbohydrates in an attempt to bring the body into serotonin balance. As a nation, we have become the most over-weight people on the face of the planet. Could it be that we all have SAD? I think not. I think it is casting too wide a net and that the real reason for the weight gain lies elsewhere.

People (those with LDIMA included) consume carbohydrates, protein and fat in excess quantity to help overcome unwelcome emotional feelings. In a similar fashion, people consume excessive amounts of caffeine to elevate their mood or alcohol to overcome shyness. These, and there are many other others, are all 'external solutions' that the mind resorts to in an attempt to avoid dealing with the essential pain of the moment.

Laurel Mellin has written a book titled 'The Solution' and created a comprehensive program designed to enable people to reprogram their neural networks by recognizing and removing the 'external solutions' they resort to in their lives in an attempt to deal with unwelcome feelings associated with unresolved emotional trash. I encourage you to visit her website. Her approach to coming to terms with undesirable emotionally sourced behavior will help you in your effort to separate what is truly an effect of light-deprivation from that of which is simply unproductive human behavior.

It has been my experience that otherwise healthy people gain weight during periods of light-deprivation either as a result of the reduction in activity that occurs naturally when you fail to recognize that seasonal or weather changes have resulted in a change in your habits; or because you are attempting to soothe unwelcome feelings. In other words, you have failed to adjust to your cessation in activity or attenuation of mood by reducing the intake of food or modifying your choices of activity, exercise or recreation.

I see no way around it. It's a 'use it or lose it' situation. Or perhaps better stated as 'move it or gain it', with the gain being weight and unwanted emotional baggage.

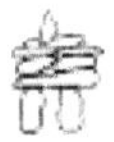

SOME HELPFUL HYPNOSIS INFORMATION

"Now you know its a meaningless question
to ask if those stories are right,
cause what matters most is the feeling
you get when you're hypnotized..."
Fleetwood Mac – 'Hypnotized'

I'd like you to think of hypnosis as a method of communication hypnotists use to create suggestibility in the mind of someone who has come seeking change or relief. You may be curious as to how this works...

Hypnotic suggestions have the power to influence behavior when the listener is:

(a) Relaxed, receptive and open to the suggestion
(b) Experiences visual, auditory, and/or kinesthetic representations of the suggestions presented

(c) Anticipates and envisions that the suggestions will result in the desired outcome(s)

Hypnosis is not mind control or brainwashing. People change their minds and actions throughout their lives. When such changes occur as a result of exposure to specific information, it is because this information has been presented through persuasion and influence. A hypnotist uses verbally expressed persuasion and influence; so do people who advertise, market goods and services; as do teachers, politicians, lawyers, entertainers, parents, and ministers.

Hypnosis may be conducted by one individual addressing another, whether in-person or through the recorded word or over the phone. You may conduct it yourself. Hypnosis fosters a greater sense of physical relaxation, with little loss of concentration or mental alertness and is often associated with being in 'trance'. Trance is a naturally occurring state in which one's attention is narrowly focused and relatively free of distractions. In fact, you may notice that hypnosis actually increases your alertness and ability to concentrate. During this process, the pressures and tension of the day will begin to disappear.

While in hypnosis, you will not become immobilized. You will remain conscious throughout and will not fall into a sleep state while under hypnosis. Even if you were to fall asleep, your mind may still continue to listen to the voice of the hypnotist. You will know exactly where you are the entire time. You may adjust your position, scratch, sneeze, or cough. You will hear with greater acuity and be generally more alert. Sounds may appear louder than usual, as your hearing may become hypersensitive while hypnotized.

Hypnosis is not sleep; instead, hypnosis puts the critical area of mind into abeyance temporarily. The critical area of mind acts like a gatekeeper to the subconscious. While hypnotized, you may still follow instructions such as moving a finger, taking a deep breath, or awakening yourself when told to do so.

There is no 'right' way to experience hypnosis. One may experience it as a deep, heavy restful feeling, while another as a light, floating sensation. Sometimes, the sensations coincide. Such is the power of suggestion. Some people hear every word spoken by the therapist, while others allow their minds to drift to other thoughts. Some experience vivid imagery, others do not. Some people remember the suggestions they hear, and some do not. Every person's experience is unique.

Hypnosis will not cause anyone to do something against their will or that contradicts their values. First, a hypnotist is ethically required to make only those suggestions that support agreed-upon outcomes. Second, clients are not receptive to suggestions that go against their morals or values—-because receptivity is one of the ingredients for success via hypnosis.

You will alert yourself and respond to any situation that needs your immediate attention. You will remain oriented as to person, place, and time.

As you enter hypnosis, certain physical changes take place within the body. You will notice your breathing becomes deeper, gentler and more rhythmic. Your lips and throat will become drier and you may develop the urge to swallow. This is normal and may be disregarded.

Hypnosis carries very few risks. Hypnosis may be contraindicated for individuals with certain medical problems, or who are actively abusing drugs or alcohol, or who are delusional or hallucinatory. Hypnosis must not be used for physical problems, such as pain, unless you have first consulted a physician to determine the underlying physical causes.

Hypnosis can be a very positive and powerful force in your life, when used wisely.

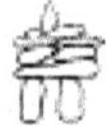

SELF-HYPNOSIS FOR LDIMA

"I hear the secrets that you keep...
when you're talking in your sleep"
The Romantics – 'Talking in Your Sleep'

By now you will be fairly familiar with hypnosis administered by another person, known as hetero-hypnosis, regardless of whether it is performed in person or by listening to a recording. I am now going to guide you through a process whereby you will take control of your own hypnotic session.

These sessions may be as brief as a few minutes or as long as you prefer to spend in trance, depending upon the amount of suggestions you wish to give yourself.

Before you begin, take a few moments to compose a laundry list of items you wish to cover once in trance, that is, improvise a hypnotic suggestion 'wish list'. It needn't be too detailed, once in trance, you will probably find you are much more focused and able to deliver them accurately, quickly and in exactly the manner you desire.

In this session you will practice a relaxation technique for a short period of time, followed by a deepening technique that is designed to take you into a safe hypnotic trance. You will count yourself into trance and then quickly administer a post-hypnotic suggestion. (Post-hypnotic suggestions are suggestions that make it easier to enter or deepen your trance the next time you practice hypnosis.) Once in trance, you will begin to recite to yourself in your mind, the suggestions you have previously decided upon in your list. Upon completing your list, you will count yourself out of trance.

It's as simple as that. A more detailed description follows with sample suggestions you may use for yourself immediately. For the sake of this sample session, I will elicit a short list of suggestions designed to help me overcome feelings of emptiness that are occurring as the days get shorter, nearer to the winter solstice. The specific behavior to influence involves impulse eating. The behavior I will substitute is a practice of deferring any and all consumption until hunger is explicitly felt.

And here we go…when you do this for real, this is the point where you normally close your eyes.

Begin by sitting upright, your back firmly against the chair, lounge or couch, with your feet up and supported by an ottoman or footrest. Remove your shoes. I want you too feel well grounded. If your arms are not supported by armrests, then place them so that your palms rest on the tops of your thighs.

Take a deep diaphragmatic breath, filling your diaphragm completely first and then fill your chest. Hold it in to a silent count of five and then exhale slowly through your mouth, pushing out all of the air by using your diaphragm again to empty all of your breath completely. Push it all out. Repeat this breath again and then again once more. After these three breaths, begin to imagine that the air is emptying out of you through the soles of your feet and as you breathe out, follow the imaginary path of your breath from the top of your head, through your chest and lower back, down through your thighs and knees, calves and ankles and then finally through the soles of your feet. Refill your belly and lungs with air once again using a diaphragmatic breath and repeat the exhalation out through the soles of your feet.

After a few more of these types of breaths, I gently ask you to visualize seeing a chalkboard in your mind. I see a black chalkboard myself, but if you prefer another color, don't let my preferences interfere with yours. As you exhale, imagine a piece of chalk is writing the following words on this chalkboard in longhand, looping the letters together as you continue to exhale to spell:

Deep Asleep

Try to work it out in your mind so that you are able to finish writing the words in the same amount of time it takes for one cycle of inhalation and exhalation. When you complete the exhalation, image the chalkboard is empty again. Don't attempt to imagine erasing it in your mind, simply see the chalkboard as empty again and repeat writing the words in longhand. At some point you will become sufficiently relaxed so that it is no longer necessary to breathe diaphragmatically and this is fine, simply let the breath go and breathe normally as you continue to visualize the words appearing in longhand on the imaginary chalkboard in your mind.

After a minute or two you will notice a sensation of drifting and you will begin to countdown slowly in your mind from twenty to zero, counting down by subtracting one with each successive count. When you reach zero say the following to yourself with a sense of urgency or self-imposed drama in your mind:

Deep Asleep!

Now immediately administer the following post-hypnotic suggestion to yourself as written below:

'Each and every time I suggest "Deep Asleep", I will sleep quickly, deeply and soundly and my physical body will relax'.

You will now be ready to recite your suggestions from the list you have previously prepared. Here's my sample list:

"I will refrain from eating until I have begun to feel the pangs of hunger. I now see myself at my perfect weight and I support myself in my efforts to attain this goal. When I feel hunger pangs, I will make healthful choices from the many wonderful foods I have purchased for myself. I will eat slowly and savor each bite and not eat any more than I feel necessary. I will defer from eating until my body tells me it needs nourishment. I will create the perfect meal for me, being careful to choose only the most nourishing and healthful foods available. This meal is the only meal that matters to me at this moment and I will create the perfect meal for myself."

Once you have completed these suggestions, you may repeat them if you so desire or begin to count yourself out of trance from one to twenty, this time by adding one to each successive count. When you reach twenty, say to yourself in your mind:

Wide Awake, now, wide-awake!

That's it! You will have completed your first self-hypnosis session. You may use this tool on the spot in your life whenever you need it, to reinforce behavioral changes. It's completely portable and best of all it's free!

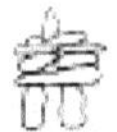

SCHEDULE WINTER BREAKS

"I want to get away, I want to fly away...yeah, yeah, yeah"
Lenny Kravitz – 'Fly Away'

One of the best things you can do to help yourself during your winter is to schedule breaks away from your light-deprived location. I like to travel to sunny, southern Florida. The accent must be on sunny. If you prefer Mexico, go for it. Almost any location significantly closer to the equator will do. Try to get at least 11 hours of sunlight if possible. I will introduce you to a website later on in the book that will help you determine the length of daylight for almost about any location on earth, any day of the year.

If you travel to the opposite hemisphere, that will be the best of all possibilities, but not really necessary. For me, Florida is good enough to return me to a 'brighter' state of mind. I begin to improve as soon as I'm out of the airline terminal at my destination; the intensity of light is so relieving.

The more often you take these 4 to 5 day mini-vacations the better. I'm writing this during one of those vacations and I have another planned for two weeks from now. As you may have already come to know, late fall through early to mid- winter are the best times for the light deprived to get away.

Florida residents have a term they use to describe the people who 'migrate' to their state during fall and winter from all parts north. They refer to them as "snowbirds". Now here's a group of highly evolved people who have a thorough understanding of what seasonal light variation is all about, even if not consciously. They truly act in their own best interest and take care of their needs. We may all learn a thing or two from the "snowbirds". If you have any of these types of people in your life, take a cue from them. As soon as they begin to make preparations to leave for Florida, you should consider starting light-therapy! If they're the real deal, upon their return, you may safely discontinue light-therapy.

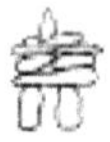

CONCLUSION

"The future's so bright, I gotta wear shades..."
Timbuk 3

Well, that's it! It's a pretty simple, yet a powerful method to banish symptoms completely. Practice it faithfully from the time you first become mindful of being light deprived and there's no reason you won't enjoy life with the same intensity as all other times of the year. You may want to share this information with the people most important to you, as they may not immediately understand why your behavior has to change so radically. They may also comment on how your schedule has become so much more structured, 'rigid' even.

If your schedule does not coincide with the rising and setting of the sun, try to schedule yourself in a manner that follows the previously suggested redefinition of a 'day'. That is, hypnosis and light-therapy before sleep and immediately upon rising.

Earlier, I mentioned that I currently reside at latitude 40. For me this means that I absolutely must practice this regimen from roughly a week or two before Thanksgiving until late February at the very minimum. I discontinued evening light-therapy sessions in late February and morning sessions in early April during the time in which I wrote the first draft of this book. It coincided with as expected, another trip to Florida, Sanibel Island specifically.

The level of cloudiness will tend to play into this equation and you may need to begin earlier depending upon that as well. I've been known to resume light therapy briefly in late April or early May because of extended rainy spells. So, think flexibly. You will eventually learn exactly what your body needs and when. Again, this is knowledge of the highest order.

You'll find references to a website in the FAQs and on the **Light Of Day** website, http://www.ldima.com that will help you to narrow down about when to start and conclude light therapy. As the day naturally lengthens, at some point you will reach a time where you may discontinue either an evening or morning light session. This is to be expected and you may observe a feeling of relief from the self-imposed structure of your day. Don't hesitate to restructure your day if and when the need arises.

As for discontinuing the use of St. John's Wort, the author recommends that you taper off the herb by cutting back over the period of a month or two. Rosenthal's book on SJW has a discussion on this and I strongly suggest you read this book thoroughly if you intend to use SJW.

I've taken prescription anti-depressants briefly in the past and experienced quite a hangover when I discontinued using them. After about four weeks I began to feel better. It was awful.

SJW may not be as difficult to withdraw from and if properly tapered, may result in little or no withdrawal effect. I know that when I alter the delivery of SJW due to vacationing in strong sunlit areas, I rarely notice that I've not taken it. I can't say the same thing when I'm up north, I can tell when it's time for another dose; especially from late fall to mid-winter.

As for the future of light therapy, I believe we've turned a corner. The future appears to belong to stronger lighting with emphasis on certain frequencies. I'm experimenting this winter with a combination blue-white light box that has twice the strength of my previous 10,000-lux box. Advanced hypnotic therapies involving regression to that younger timeframe when you first became susceptible may provide a greater level of comfort above and beyond the already effective relief the hypnosis I enthusiastically recommend provides. I will be scheduling a session or two with my hypnotherapist over the phone to do some regression therapy to try to find out if it is possible to locate a past source of beliefs that may be contributing to my situation. Respect for the power of hypnosis and NLP techniques have become accepted into the mainstream of modern day life.

I'm curious to know if my metabolic type has any relation to LDIMA. Could a diet component be added to the mix? Why not? If so, what will it look like?

I am currently enrolled in the Solution, a program where you retrain your neural networks for health and happiness. You can find a link to it on the Light of Day website http://www.ldima.com. I'm hoping to find that SJW is just another external solution that can be safely left behind.

Until then, live each and every day to its fullest potential. I thank you for taking the time to review this material.

Before I leave you, there are some things you can do today to start you on your journey to year-round wholeness. Get a blank journal. Begin to note your level of effectiveness daily. Often just taking this step to write things down encourages you to do what will empower you.

Visit and bookmark the websites I've mentioned so that you can find out what the degradation curve of daylight looks like for your city.

Get yourself a good quality hypnotic recording and begin to listen to it first thing in the morning, every day. Make this your special time, just for you.

Do some research on light boxes. Become more knowledgeable on the options available. If the budget is tight, consider a used light box Build onto what you have learned today and make it a habit to add to that every day.

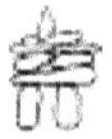

FAQS

In my 'day' job, I supervise a team of Human Resources focused Information Technology analysts for a major health care products company as they support global web applications; think baby powder and you have a pretty good idea what company I'm referring to.

Part of my job is to manage the content of a self-service support website, so I'm no stranger to frequently asked questions. If you're here you've probably already read through the material above so I'll keep this short and to the point.

Q. How can I tell if I have LDIMA?

A. If you experience a significant decline in mood the closer you get to the winter solstice, and spontaneously recover completely by the time of the summer solstice, you almost certainly have LDIMA.

Q. In real-time, what does LDIMA feel like?

A. Let me give you a few examples of how I know when I am light deprived, hopefully without going too deeply into any of them.

The first is the unprovoked sensation that something is missing and an accompanying feeling of dread that seems to come out of nowhere. Another is the experience of so-called 'morning depression' which is really nothing more than a sluggishness upon awakening that is reluctant to abate in late fall or early to mid-winter. It kind of feels like a hangover, except that you haven't had any alcohol.

Another is the tendency to question what I've recently concluded as reasonable and sound ideas and plans, often within the same day. So an idea conceived during the daytime, seems deficient later in the evening, after darkness has set in. Still another is when I simply can't seem to make up my mind on something or have difficulty with seemingly simple decisions, or worse still, flip-flopping back and forth on relatively insignificant decisions, like what to wear for example.

Another example and this is very telling…is to travel to the lighting department of your local Home Depot or any lighting store for that matter. If you notice your mood begins to improve the longer you stand there (and don't be bashful, walk around and pretend you are comparing lighting for that eventual upgrade you'll no doubt be making in your home), you're a candidate for light supplementation.

If you become dreary-minded on cloudy, snowy, or rainy late fall days and perk up on subsequent bright and sunny days, you are very close to a diagnosis. This will not happen to me in June or July, but in August or September, look out!

Another way I know I am susceptible from light deprivation is what I call the 'road kill' indicator. During the summer, when I pass a dead deer or other wild animal that is certainly not anyone's pet, I have this feeling that it is normal and all part of the natural order of things. But during late fall and early winter, when I begin to feel morbid over seeing this, I know I need to take care of myself and begin to get or make plans for some light supplementation.

Q. I've been told that people with LDIMA tend to gain weight during winter. Is that a symptom?

A. Weight gain is a bogus issue as far as LDIMA is concerned. I've found that it occurs because you are not getting the same level of movement and exercise you normally do during the more active times of the year. Thanksgiving, Christmas and New Years bring additional opportunities to consume without adequate time for purging the excess. Wear a pedometer in summer and winter and check for yourself. Craving carbohydrates such as sweets is another bogus issue and best dealt with independently of light-deprivation.

If you're having problems with eating, check out the excellent book by Laurel Mellin titled 'The Solution', I believe you will find excessive consumption is emotionally related. But please finish this one first…you're so close anyway. I chose to include suggestions for controlling 'food cravings' in the chapter on self-hypnosis because it is a topic we can easily relate to and you will be able to see significant progress almost immediately, regardless of the time of year, even if you do not have LDIMA.

Q. Why use light-therapy?

A. Light therapy does two things for you. It artificially lengthens the day for your brain, reducing the level of mood attenuation in the process by stimulating the production of serotonin and reducing the production of melatonin. In other words, it works to correct the source of the problem.

Q. What's a light-box?

A. It's a box with light in it...I'm kidding! In my job, I don't get to be funny in the Q&A section of our website so please indulge me here. A light-box is a strong light intended to recreate the natural sensation of the sun as it shines on your face. A good light-box will emit light rays that cover the full-spectrum of visible light, minus the harmful ultra-violet rays.

Q. Must I use stronger lighting in my home?

A. Absolutely. When I moved into a new home a couple years ago, one of the first things I did (I moved in October, so I knew time was of the essence), was to systematically upgrade each rooms lighting to allow for the possibility of very bright lighting. For example, my master bathroom now has a light strip with 8 40-watt clear rounds bulbs in it and it has a mirror background for maximum reflection. When I purchased the home, it had one sixty-watt bulb in a milky diffused bathroom fixture. When I get up in the morning, the lights go on and it gets bright in a hurry and I become functional very rapidly. The so-called 'morning depression' quickly becomes a thing of the past.

Q. Why all the emphasis on hypnosis?

A. Hypnosis replaces the awkward feeling of being different from everyone else and restores self-esteem and self-confidence. It takes repetition to become fully effective. Think of it like working out for your mind. It can also help you in other areas of your life and when the time comes to discontinue light therapy, you may choose to continue on with the hypnosis. It can be applied successfully in many areas of your life in addition to overcoming the unwelcome feelings that coincide with light-deprivation. There's an abundance of hypnosis recordings available for every conceivable topic. Don't listen to hypnosis recordings while driving.

Q. I understand that I need to have my eyes open to receive the maximum benefit from light therapy. Is that true?

A. No, absolutely not. Eyes closed are equally as good if not safer. I suggest that you experiment with shining it on the undersides of your knees or knee pits if you will, I've found it to be effective there as well. Think of all the people you see lying on the beach face down with their feet up in the air exposing the backs of their legs to the sun. It feels good and there must be something more to it than tanning. The nerves that carry impulses to the pineal gland travel through the back of the neck, it may be helpful to shine bright light there as well.

Q. I'm afraid to take Saint John's Wort, can I get addicted to it?

A. St. John's Wort functions as an herbal anti-depressant. You may become accustomed to feeling well, with the only side effect of discontinuing use being the possibility of not feeling as well as you did before. It is gentle with few, if any, side effects. Please consult your physician if you are currently taking another medication in response to a diagnosis of depression. Please read Rosenthal's book, SJW – The Herbal Way to Feeling Good.

Q. Why take such a massive dose of vitamin D?

A. I had a blood test taken one winter and the doctor was very concerned with the lowness of my vitamin D level. At the time I was taking 400 IU of cholecalciferol 4 times a day and still did not get my count up. So for convenience sake, the 50,000 iu dosage was prescribed. Originally, I took it daily, but after a retest, it was discovered that I was over-saturated and needed to discontinue taking it until I got back to normal. We settled on once a week starting late-fall and continuing through the winter.

Q. Why does the author like trance music?

A. The idea is to more naturally stimulate your heart to beat at a faster pace to enhance feelings of motivation and inspiration. If you exercise by running in the winter, you may be able to do that, but I'm expecting lots of people to be limited by their environment and trance music has the right number of beats per minute. If you play drums, try that. If you want more of a benefit, play trance music loud, in your music player of choice, if necessary.

Q. Can I get the same benefit as light therapy from visiting a tanning salon?

A. I honestly don't know, sorry. Concentrated exposure to UV light sounds very dangerous.

Q. I don't know if I can take the schedule, it seems like a large investment of time, is there any way around that?

A. Short of moving south, I haven't an answer. You have to restore the length of daylight. However you are able to do that in a manner that works for you is what's absolutely necessary to obtain a complete recovery. I found that getting only light-therapy was not enough. I needed the hypnosis to completely restore the feeling of wellness I experience in the month of June. The old saw, "once begun, half done" rings true for light therapy and hypnosis; except this therapy is 'effortless'. All you have to do is close your eyes and listen.

Q. How long will it take before I begin to feel results?

A. That will vary from individual to individual. Initially, depending upon when you begin treatment, it may take a week or two depending upon how light-deprived you are at the point in time. Once you have become conditioned to it, you may begin to feel better almost immediately.

My first experience using the light-box only was that it was four days before I began to feel anything resembling normalcy. I am now able to restore this feeling in a day or two. The hypnosis has somewhat more than an additive effect; its effects are of a more lasting nature.

Q. How can I approximate the amount of light therapy needed to restore well being?

A. I recently completed a four-night trip to Fort Myers Beach, which accomplished the goal of eliminating symptoms, even if only briefly, as it always will. This is the only true way I know of to test yourself to see if you have LDIMA. Upon my return, I wanted to determine how much supplemental light therapy would be needed. The good folks at ptaff.ca have a handy web page that will generate graphs that can be used to determine this. Here's the URL: http://ptaff.ca/soleil/?lang=en_CA
If you look below you will see a graph I generated that shows the sunrise, sunset and total daylight for my hometown of Somerset, NJ. Below it, you will find a similar graph for Fort Myers, where I recently vacationed. You can see that the total amount of daylight differs by 1:05.

Assuming I felt complete relief after the four-days. It is reasonable to expect that no more than about an hour of light therapy will be needed to maintain a level of complete relief. In actuality, the amount of light therapy needed will continue to decline as the amount

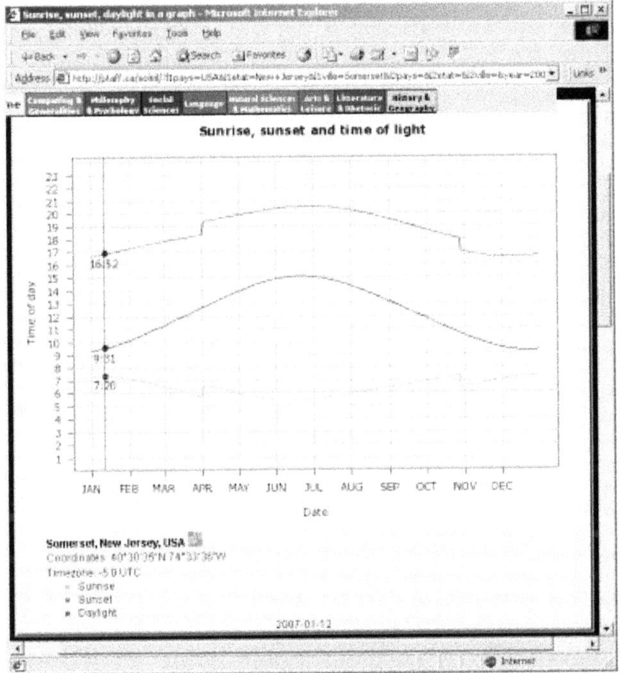
Sunrise, sunset, daylight in a graph - Microsoft Internet Explorer
Sunrise, sunset and time of light
Time of day
16:52
7:20
JAN
FEB
MAR
APR
MAY
JUN
JUL
AUG
SEP
OCT
NOV
DEC
Date
Somerset, New Jersey, USA
Timezone: -5.0 UTC
Sunrise
Sunset
Daylight
2007-01-12

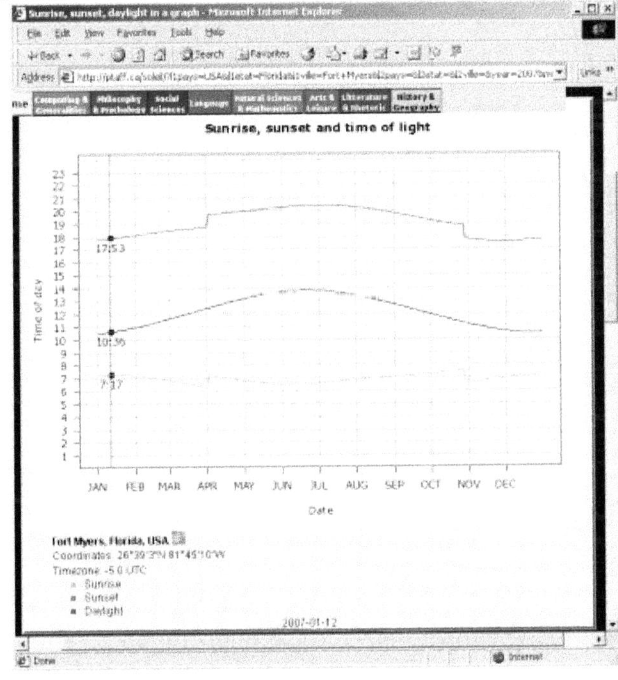
Sunrise, sunset, daylight in a graph - Microsoft Internet Explorer
Sunrise, sunset and time of light
Time of day
17:53
10:36
7:17
JAN
FEB
MAR
APR
MAY
JUN
JUL
AUG
SEP
OCT
NOV
DEC
Date
Fort Myers, Florida, USA
Timezone: -5.0 UTC
Sunrise
Sunset
Daylight
2007-01-12

of natural daylight lengthens. It is also reasonable to expect that I can consider terminating light therapy when the amount of daylight at Somerset, NJ meets or exceeds 10:36 minutes, give or take a few minutes.

I haven't completely found that to be true for me. I work indoors and will need to get outdoors more to completely eliminate light therapy once the length of day exceed 10 hours and 36 minutes, as in the previous example. Cloudiness may interfere with the best of plans; so let your feelings guide you.

Q. I'm on a limited budget, how would you implement the program given strict limitations on spending.

A. Unfortunately, for me it was never enough simply using light-therapy. That's why the caption on the inside cover states 'Light+Hypnosis+Herbs+Trance'. I believe the order in which I presented them is the correct order. If I were to hedge on the specific order, it will be between hypnosis and herbs, perhaps they may be switched, depending upon the severity of symptoms. But on a limited budget, the initial order presented is how I will choose to spend my money.

If you can reliably obtain strong sunlight daily, you can forego purchasing a light-box. Indoor home lighting will never resemble anything close to 10,000 lux. A light-box can be had for two hundred dollars and it is money well spent and perhaps reimbursable through your health plan. A hypnosis recording can be found for under $20. SJW is going to be the most expen-

> sive part of the treatment over the long run. I suggest you hold off on going that route to see if you are able to make a significant recovery happen for you without using the herbs. Trance music is like icing on the cake and is really intended to strengthen you quickly once a solid foundation has been built. It makes a great pick-me-up at any time of the day or night. Trance music recordings are inexpensive and can be obtained used.

Okay, I think that covers most of the concerns people will have that are considering this…I wish you all the best. Remember, if you truly are a light-deprived person, even if you do nothing, your situation is bound to improve as the day naturally lengthens. My hope is that you will take as much action as necessary to eliminate your symptoms whenever they appear.

Ideally speaking, once you have confirmed to yourself that you are light deprived, it stands to reason that relocation to a place where you will never experience less than your minimum daily requirement of daylight is the correct solution. It isn't that easy a decision for everyone.

If you follow these suggestions, I believe you will come to learn a great deal more about your mindbody connection. You will be able to predict and react in a fashion that completely mitigates the symptoms of LDIMA…and once you have this power, it will be yours for as long as you need it.

Be well!

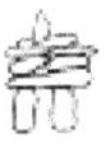

SUGGESTED READING

Light, Medicine of the Future by Jacob Liberman O.D. Ph.D., Bear & Company Inc., Santa Fe, NM 87504-2860

Professional Hypnotism Manual by John G. Kappas Ph.D., Panorama Publishing Co. (800) 634-5620

St. John's Wort: The Miracle Cure for Depression by Norman Rosenthal M.D., HarperCollins Publishers

The Pathway by Laurel Mellin, ReganBooks - Harper Collins Publishers Inc., New York, NY

APPENDIX OF HELPFUL WEBSITES

Light of Day website

http://www.ldima.com

St. John's Wort and Sun Don't Mix

http://www.fordham.edu/campus_resources/public_affairs/archives/2000/archive_208.asp

Sunrise/Sunset Table for US and locations worldwide

http://aa.usno.navy.mil/data/docs/RS_OneYear.html
(there are no dropdowns for city names, so please experiment to find a location close to yours)

Sunrise, sunset, daylight in a graph

http://ptaff.ca/soleil/?lang=en_CA

The Mental Bank Concept

http://www.hypnosis.edu/streaming/mental-bank/

The Solution

http://www.thepathway.org

Seasonal Affective Disorder is depression

http://www.upi.com/ConsumerHealthDaily/view.php?StoryID=20070126-062353-4967r

(this article is reprinted below in its entirety)

ROCHESTER, N.Y., Jan. 26 (UPI) — A University of Rochester research review says that Seasonal Affective Disorder is actually a subtype of major depression and should be treated as such.

Lead author Dr. Stephen Lurie, an assistant professor of family medicine at the University of Rochester Medical Center, said that SAD is sometimes missed in the typical doctor's office setting.

"Like major depression, Seasonal Affective Disorder probably is under-diagnosed in primary care offices," Lurie said. "But with personalized and detailed attention to symptoms, most patients can be helped a great deal."

For some patients, SAD is precipitated by darker days causing a shift in 24-hour hormonal rhythms. The loss of natural light outdoors can be replaced with treatment by indoor light-therapy units designed for SAD. Light therapy is best delivered in the morning, when it can regulate the daily pattern of melatonin secretion, according to the review published in the American Academy of Family Physicians.

www.ingramcontent.com/pod-product-compliance
Ingram Content Group UK Ltd.
Pitfield, Milton Keynes, MK11 3LW, UK
UKHW020139250726
13967UKWH00002B/757